7/05

DATE DUE

AUG 10			

WRITTEN IN FRUSTRATION

WRITTEN IN FRUSTRATION

JACK DREYFUS

Lantern Books • New York
A Division of Booklight Inc.

2005
Lantern Books
One Union Square West, Suite 201
New York, NY 10003

Copyright Jack Dreyfus 2005

Printed in the United States of America

This book is dedicated to
Mark Twain, to Helen Raudonat,
to Joan Personette, and to Johnny.

CONTENTS

Part Two: Probabilities

Part Three: Worcester County Jail Study

Part Four: Experiences

Part Five: Conclusion

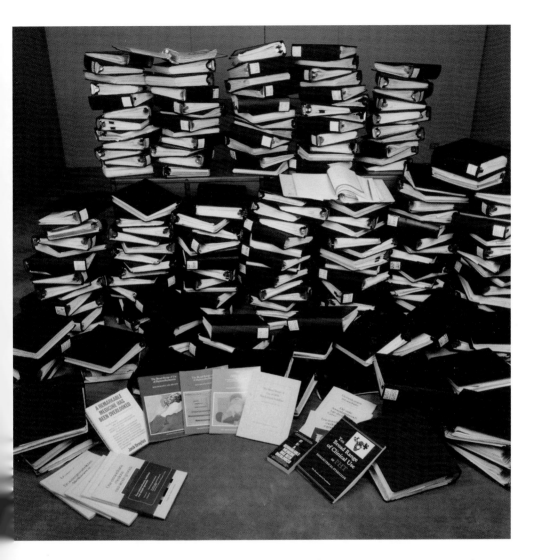

A photograph of over 10,000 studies from 38 countries, published in over 250 medical journals, detailing studies on Dilantin (phenytoin). This picture was taken in 1984.

A 2001 picture of over 23,000 studies from 48 countries, published in over 350 medical journals, is on the next page. A collection of works by Jack Dreyfus and the Dreyfus Medical Foundation is on page xii.

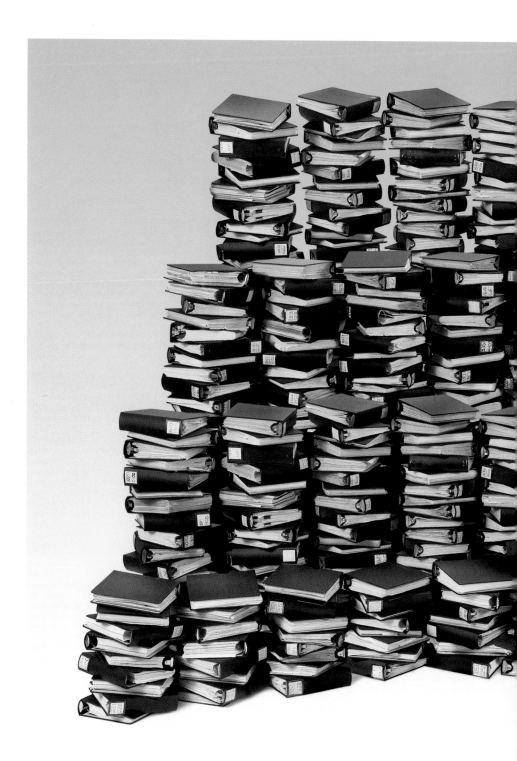

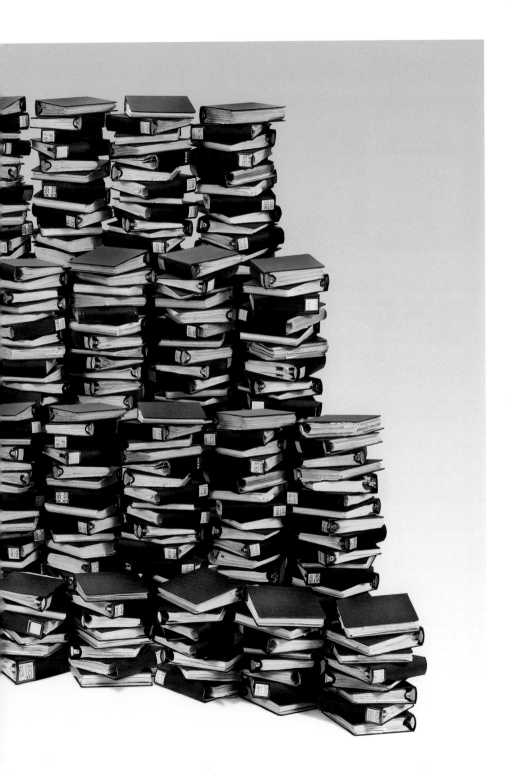

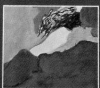

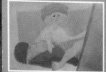

INTRODUCTION

I WAS FORTY-FIVE YEARS OLD AND HAD BEEN SEE-ing Dr. Max Silbermann, a fine psychiatrist, for four-and-a-half years, six days a week, to talk about my mostly imagined problems. I had an endogenous (coming from within) depression.

One night, I asked Max if he would let me try phenytoin (Dilantin), the drug given to epileptics. He did, and, overnight, I was well.

Could this medicine help others as it helped me?

After unsuccessful attempts to get the medical profession to investigate, I resigned as President of the Dreyfus Fund and Senior Partner of Dreyfus and Company—two highly successful businesses—-and established the Dreyfus Medical Foundation.

Over the years, the Foundation's research library

discovered an increasing amount of studies published in over 350 medical journals, from forty-eight countries, written in twenty different languages, reporting phenytoin to be useful for more than eighty symptoms and disorders. The Foundation condensed these studies into bibliographies, one in 1970, another in 1975, and a third in 1988, and sent them to all the physicians in the United States. The 1988 edition contained 3,100 medical references, and was accompanied by a book, *A Remarkable Medicine Has Been Overlooked*, which I had written.

President John F. Kennedy said, "Ask not what your country can do for you—ask what you can do for your country." However, I've found that giving a gift to my country is not easy. I brought this information to two Presidents (attempted to meet with two others) and four Secretaries of Health, three Commissioners of the FDA, one Surgeon General, and a host of senators, congressmen, and physicians. Still, nothing official has happened.

Recently, I met with seventy-three physicians from the following countries: Brazil, Bulgaria, Cameroon, China, Dominican Republic, El Salvador, Ghana, Guyana, India, Indonesia, Jordan, Lithuania, Mali, Nigeria, Poland, Romania, Slovakia, Tanzania,

United Kingdom, Uganda, Ukraine, and Zambia. Each of these countries gave me gifts and compliments. I appreciated the gifts, but told them the compliments were due to phenytoin.

To a large extent, due to the Foundation's efforts, phenytoin (also known as PHT) is now being used in Russia, China, Ghana, India, and Mexico for an ever-increasing number of symptoms and disorders. Although phenytoin was introduced in the United States in 1938, its only listing with the FDA is for a single disorder. Many millions in this country suffer, needlessly.

The contents of this book, *Written in Frustration*, are pieces that I've written in my frustration over the years. I put this together with the hope that it will influence you to study the evidence found in my fourth book, *The Story of a Remarkable Medicine*.

Good Health and Good Luck,

Jack Dreyfus

PART ONE

Written in Frustration

1. BLANK PIECE OF PAPER

TAKE A PIECE OF BLANK PAPER, A LARGE PIECE, and put it in your head in the section where you keep your "knowledge." Don't, at this time, let any of your "knowledge" get on it.

In 1906, the FDA was established by Congress. It was given certain specific obligations. It's obvious that Congress could not see into the long-term future all the ramifications. But it's clear that Congress established the FDA to help with the health of the American public. If you don't believe this, you can put the blank piece of paper in the bathroom, near the toilet, where it can be useful. If you do believe the FDA was established to help with the health of the American public, we will start with a story.

In 1908, a German chemist, Heinrich Biltz, synthesized a substance, diphenylhydantoin. He sold it to a drug company named Parke-Davis. Parke-Davis tested it on six healthy mice and, not observing any changes, decided that the substance was not useful. It sat on their shelves for the next twenty-nine years, while the patents expired.

In 1938, two physicians, outside of Parke-Davis, were looking for a better anti-epileptic drug than phenobarbital. Phenobarbital was effective, but it was also a sedative, and not as effective as was desirable.

Drs. Putnam and Merritt didn't have epileptic animals, so they constructed a box in which they put cats and jolted the cats with electricity. After enough electricity had been received, the cats had convulsions. Of twenty-five drugs which were tried, diphenylhydantoin (phenytoin) was, by far, the most effective in preventing these convulsions. Since Putnam and Merritt were looking for an anti-epileptic, it's natural that they would say, "Eureka, we have an anti-epileptic drug," and they did.

But Putnam and Merritt also had a drug that was effective against inappropriate electricity. At that time, it was not well-known that most of the body's functions are bio-electrically motivated. Putnam and Merritt had found a drug with enormous potential.

Phenytoin was tried on the epileptics. It was far more effective than phenobarbital, and it was given to people with intractable epilepsy, with good results. Also, it did not have the sedative effects of phenobarbital.

What's more, not only did phenytoin not have the negative effects of phenobarbital, it had positive effects. A few months after it was used on the epileptics, physicians started to report that the people who'd received it had improvement in personality, mood, memory, concentration, and amenability to discipline. This had not happened with phenobarbital. So, this was, in effect, a controlled study, phenobarbital having been used as a control.

From that point on, physicians throughout the world gradually started using phenytoin for an ever-increasing number of symptoms and disorders, other than epilepsy.

One must consider, there are 3,400 medical journals in the world; the average physician receives seven or eight. If he reads all of them, thoroughly, he will have less than one-half of one percent of the world literature. Further, the studies on phenytoin have been reported from forty-eight countries and written in twenty different languages, so it's obvious the physicians couldn't know all of the work of the others. The work that was reported was reported in over 350 medical journals, and we must keep in mind that medical journals do not accept just "any study." They require a certain degree of apparent reliability.

Since it was impossible for most of these physicians to know the work of others, their work had the most compelling independence and objectivity possible. These physicians were not paid by drug companies to make these reports. They did it with one thing in mind: to help people.

Let's shift for a moment and go to the question of how a physician becomes aware of drugs that are therapeutic for the symptoms that he encounters. In our system, they are brought to him by the drug companies, through advertisements, and by their salesmen. If the physician does not learn about a drug in this fashion, he just doesn't think about it. I'm not saying all physicians, but most physicians. Further, for the last twenty-five years, there's been a rotten procedure by some lawyers who sue physicians just to get settlements, whether there's any merit, or non-merit, in the suits. So, physicians have learned to be careful, and hospital committees have been careful to do things in a standard way.

When their drug was found useful in 1938, Parke-Davis sold it for a penny per 100-mg capsule. It didn't occur to them that phenytoin was useful for anything else. But even when it did occur to them, they didn't think of bringing it to the FDA because of the millions of dollars it would cost to have it approved, and the time that would have to be spent. So, it lay there, ignored by the drug company because it was out of patent. And, for the same financial reasons, no other drug company saw fit to bring it to the FDA.

The evidence that Parke-Davis has known about phenytoin's many uses is extensive, in writing, and can be shown when the time is appropriate.

In 1972, four physicians, and Dr. Charles Edwards, Commissioner of the FDA, attended a two-day conference at the offices of the Dreyfus Medical Foundation on the subject of phenytoin. As a result of that meeting, Dr. Edwards said he didn't know what he could do because he was used to a drug company bringing applications to the FDA, but he had an idea. If the Dreyfus Foundation could get a responsible political figure to write a letter to HEW Secretary Elliot Richardson, they could have Secretary Richardson write an appropriate letter that would be useful. Governor Rockefeller wrote such a letter, and

Secretary Richardson wrote the following (excerpt):

June 12, 1972

Dear Governor Rockefeller:

Please forgive the delay of this response to your April 19th letter concerning the current status of the drug, phenytoin.

Conversations with health officials within the Department have revealed that phenytoin (PHT) was introduced in 1938 as the first essentially non-sedating anti-convulsant drug. The dramatic effect of PHT and its widespread acceptance in the treatment of convulsive disorders may have tended to obscure a broader range of therapeutic uses.

A review of the literature reveals that phenytoin has been reported to be useful in a wide range of disorders. Among its reported therapeutic actions are its stabilizing effect on the nervous system, its anti-arrhythmic effect on certain cardiac disorders, and its therapeutic effect on emotional disorders.

The fact that such broad therapeutic effects

have been reported by many independent scientists and physicians over a long period of time would seem to indicate that the therapeutic effects of phenytoin are more than that of an anti-convulsant.

The FDA encourages the submission of formal applications which, of course, would include the necessary supporting evidence for the consideration of approval for a wider range of therapeutic uses.

Your interest in encouraging the Department to provide a *public clarification** of the status of phenytoin is very welcome, and I hope this information is responsive to your concerns.

With warm regards,
Sincerely,

Elliot L. Richardson

*Note: Our emphasis. Secretary Richardson said this letter could be made public.

Here we have a drug that's been reported to be useful by independent and objective physicians for more than eighty symptoms and disorders. It's a drug whose

safety has been explored more extensively than, perhaps, any other drug. For over sixty years, millions of
people have taken it every day. Thus, it has had the
most extensive and intensive test of its safety. It's not
on the list of controlled drugs because it's non-habit
forming. In some countries, it's not even a prescrip-
tion drug.

The negative side effects of phenytoin are few and
not serious. If one is allergic, one can't take it (an estimated three percent of the population). A much small-
er percent don't metabolize it properly and may have
to take small amounts or none at all. With infected
gums (not healthy gums), phenytoin's ability to heal
can cause hypertrophy.

The beneficial side effects are many, and extremely
valuable. Even a cursory study of *The Story of a
Remarkable Medicine*'s cardiac section, the section on
anti-anoxic effects, phenytoin's salutary effects on
high-density lipoproteins, and its effects on stress,
shows that phenytoin is a substance with protective
effects, and coins the phrase, "beneficial side effects."

We're sympathetic with the Food and Drug
Administration up to a point. They don't have an arm
to go out and search for the work of physicians around
the world. But, in this case, it's been done for them.

Independent physicians have spent millions of hours studying this. Because of an extraordinary piece of luck, the Dreyfus Medical Foundation learned that phenytoin was more than an anti-convulsant and has gathered this information from around the world for the FDA.

Still, the physician waits for the FDA to do something, and the absence of their doing something makes him feel that there must be something wrong. Besides, many physicians have long ago gotten over the habit of reading things that are not absolutely necessary. So, to some extent, the evidence, even though it's been sent to all the physicians, is being ignored. The FDA has made it clear that an unapproved use does not mean a disapproved use. If a drug has been approved for safety, a doctor may use it as he sees fit. Nevertheless, there's that legal fear that the doctors, understandably, have.

Now, we have a most unusual condition. We have a drug reported to be useful all over the world for the widest variety of disorders, and the FDA has it listed for only a single disorder, namely epilepsy. This limited listing is ridiculous, and causes great harm. But now that the world literature has been collected for them, we believe the FDA would like to do something to correct this.

Whether they should take this matter use by use and approve it for one thing after another is questionable; that could take forever. However, the FDA could say in the package insert:

> In this rare and unusual case, a drug was out of patent before it was discovered useful for anything, and, as a result, the parenting company has done nothing to bring other uses to the FDA's attention.
>
> We feel it's our responsibility to make you aware that doctors around the world have published thousands of papers, in over 350 medical journals, reporting it useful for a wide variety of disorders. We refer the physician to his medical literature.
>
> We remind the physician of what was said in our 1982 Bulletin:
>
> *The Federal Food, Drug, and Cosmetic Act does not limit the manner in which a physician may use an approved drug. Once a product has been approved for marketing, a physician may prescribe it for uses, or in treatment regimens, or patient populations,*

that are not included in approved labeling. Such "unapproved" or, more precisely, "unlabeled" uses may, in fact, reflect approaches to drug therapy that have been extensively reported in medical literature.

Now that this blank piece of paper has been filled in, you can allow your present "knowledge" to accept it.

2. THE TUNA FISH STORY

ONCE UPON A TIME, SOME PEOPLE WERE SHIP-wrecked on a desert island. Their only food was tiny fish they caught daily. To get the most from the fish they constructed a machine that ground them up, including the heads and tails.

A year went by, and all the food the people ate went through the machine. Five years went by, ten years, and still their food went through the machine.

One day, a man caught a tuna. "Now we will all have plenty to eat," he said.

"Put it through the machine," the people told him.

"It's too big," he said, "it won't fit."

"Then we can't eat it," they said.

Like the tuna fish story, the phenytoin story is too big. It won't fit in the FDA machine.

—Jonas, "The Soft Robot"

13

3. THE GREAT DANE
AND THE CRICKET

DURING THE MID-1960S, AS I SAW MORE AND more evidence of the usefulness of phenytoin (PHT), I buttonholed any doctor I ran into and informally talked about PHT. I invited some doctors—Dr. Steiner and Dr. Klarch (fictitious names)—to dinner to discuss it. I appreciated their time was valuable and told them they could bill me for it. Dr. Steiner didn't send a bill. Dr. Klarch sent a bill for $500. This seemed high. His only contribution to the meeting had been "Please pass the butter."

I must have spoken to dozens of doctors during this period. None of them had heard of PHT being used for anything other than epilepsy. They were all (with one exception) polite, even kind, but they didn't give

me any encouragement. One doctor looked at me the
way a Great Dane looks at a cricket and explained:
"Medicine is a complicated matter, and I'd advise you
to stick to Wall Street."

Bless his heart.

4. HIS SATANIC MAJESTY

IN MY BOOK, A REMARKABLE MEDICINE HAS BEEN *Overlooked*, I said, "If you want the government to do something outside of routine, and expect to see it happen in your lifetime, you'd better arrange for reincarnation."

On my 80th birthday, I sent in an application for reincarnation. The next day, His Satanic Majesty appeared and said my application had been turned down. But he was friendly, and told me an air-conditioned condominium had been reserved for me. I expressed appreciation.

Then I asked if Dr. Blank* and Dr. Blankest* of the FDA were going to be down there. Satan's tail wriggled a bit, and he said, "I have to draw the line somewhere."

*Real names weren't used; I didn't want Satan to be sued.

5. WALKING BY A LAKE

LET US START WITH AN ANALOGY. TWO MEN ARE walking along the side of a lake. "A" will profit by "B's" death. Knowing "B" can't swim, he pushes him into the lake, and "B" drowns. Our laws say this is murder, punishable by death.

Or, "A" and "B" are walking along the side of a lake. "A" will profit by "B's" death. "B" slips and falls into the lake. A life preserver is nearby that "A" could throw to save "B's" life. He doesn't, and "B" drowns. Is there anything wrong with this? Our laws don't say so, but the Lord does.

Millions of people have slipped into the lake, and Parke-Davis hasn't even tried to throw them a life preserver; the FDA says it's none of their business. Is

there anything wrong with this? The devil doesn't
think so.

6. OUR FILE CARDS ARE SPILLED ON THE FLOOR

The greatest crisis facing us is a crisis in the organization and accessibility of human knowledge. We own an enormous "encyclopedia" which isn't even arranged alphabetically. Our "file cards" are spilled on the floor. The answers we want may be buried somewhere in the heap.—Robert Heinlein

THE OUTSTANDING SCIENCE FICTION WRITER Robert Heinlein made this brilliant observation. It describes what has happened with phenytoin.

The encyclopedia of human knowledge about this drug has been scattered around the world. Thousands of independent and objective physicians, not sponsored by a drug company, have reported in over 350 medical journals, written in twenty different languages, that phenytoin is useful for over eighty symptoms and disorders. When this information had been looked for, translated into one language, and summarized into bibliographies, as it was by the Dreyfus Medical Foundation, the "file cards" were no longer buried in the heap.

Aesop's fables would not have lasted this long if they didn't have merit. The story of the boy who cried wolf is applicable here. So many "miracle drugs" and "wonder drugs" have been tested and found lacking that when a real wolf, in this case a pack of wolves, comes along, the reading of the evidence is ignored by most.

7. WILL THE SUN RISE?

IF IT WERE ESSENTIAL FOR THE HEALTH OF THE American public to have it listed with the FDA that the sun will rise in the East, this would not be achieved overnight.

After all, we have only the anecdotal evidence from numerous independent observers, the theories of astronomers. But, who knows, perhaps the Almighty may put the cosmos into reverse tomorrow to keep the parts from wearing out? Perhaps.

No, the proposition would have to go through the routine review procedures of the FDA, and this would take time.

8. BUSY

YEARS AGO, I TRIED TO INTEREST A PRESIDENtial candidate in this great, overlooked medicine. He told me he was too busy. This made me think of the word busy and what it means. I think a good definition is:

The amount of time spent, multiplied by the importance of the thing it's spent on.

About sixty years ago, in a convalescent camp in the Coast Guard, I was given a stick with a nail on the end of it to pick up cigarette butts to keep me busy. I was not too conscientious, but we won the war anyway.

9. THE SUPREME COURT

To become a member of the Supreme Court a candidate is put through many weeks of grueling questioning by Congressmen. Congress knows all the members of the Supreme Court, and almost none of the members of the FDA. We have a strange situation here. If the Supreme Court makes a dumb ruling, and I don't say they do, there would be a public outcry, because we would all know about it. If the FDA does something dumb, and I do say they do, the public says, "It must be so, the FDA said so."

10. THE CAVES
OF KNOWLEDGE

WHEN SOMETHING THAT'S NEVER HAPPENED, never came close to happening, does happen, it follows that there are skeptics galore. The knowledge that it can't happen is enclosed in the "Caves of Knowledge."

I have never read anything on the subject of how we remember. However, it appears that when we are satisfied we know something, we put it in a little cave in our brain and cover the front with cement so we won't lose it. Otherwise, we would have to learn things over and over again; our brains would be in chaos.

If phenytoin is not a benign and remarkably versatile medicine, how else can one explain the following?

In 1975 IMS America, Ltd. did a study of the symptoms and disorders for which physicians in the U.S. used a variety of drugs. The list of the uses of phenytoin is included here:

anti-convulsant

prophylaxis

cardiac arrhythmias

anti-coagulant

pain relief

control heart rate

relieve headache

withdrawal symptoms

analgesic

psychotherapeutic

control dizziness

anti-neuritic

reduce tension

relieve migraine

sedative/promote sleep

stimulant

tranquilizer

anti-nausea

uterine sedative

anti-depressant

anti-spasmodic

mood elevation

anti-allergic

migraines

control vertigo

GI anti-spasmodic

anti-hemorrhagic

cardiotonic

The most compelling evidence is the fact that phenytoin, introduced in the United States, is now being used for over fifty symptoms and disorders in Russia, China, Ghana, India, and Mexico.

The safety of phenytoin has probably had the most

extensive testing of any drug. For more than sixty years, millions of people have taken it daily. Its chief negative side effect (an allergic reaction) is a rash which occurs in an estimated three percent of the population. Phenytoin is not habit forming and it has many beneficial side effects.

When a drug has been reported useful for over eighty symptoms and disorders it is almost impossible to believe. One has to remove the cement from the Caves of Knowledge. Use dynamite, if necessary.

11. SUGGESTION FOR CONGRESS AND THE AMERICAN PEOPLE

MANY YEARS AGO, WHEN I READ THAT MARK Twain said, "Government is organized imbecility," I thought he was being humorous. I don't think so anymore.

For nearly forty years, I've been trying to give the United States government a great present, but I've found that there's no place in government for presents; there are plenty of places to receive problems. However, I don't think we should pick on the politicians about this, I think we should pick on ourselves; at least as much as on them.

Congress and the President are supposed to have the most important jobs in the United States; they run our country. We should pay them top salaries, and we don't even come close. Our Senators get $150,000, plus perks; the same for Congressmen. Our President gets $400,000, plus perks.

The average major league baseball player (there are 700 of them) receives about $1.2 million a year. In other words, the average baseball player earns eight times as much as a member of Congress, and three times as much as our Chief Executive Officer, the President of the United States.

Here are some annual earnings of recent date:

Top CEOs (in millions):
$141.1, 74.8, 70.5, 54.4, 54.1, 52.9, 45.8, 40.6, 36.1, 35.9

—Business Week

Top Athletes (in millions):
$80.3, 42.0, 35.0, 31.9, 29.7, 28.2, 26.2, 26.1, 25.9, 23.2

—Forbes

I won't give you any more figures. You'll find them in the sports pages every day.

SUGGESTION

Let's pay our Senators $3.5 million; members of the House $3.5 million; the President $7.5 million. If you say they're not worth it, that may be so. But that's just the point. If we pay outstanding salaries in government, maybe we'll get outstanding people. Compared to our national debt of $7.5 trillion, this is peanuts.

PART TWO

Probabilities

12. THE LION STORY

YOU HAVE A FIRST-FLOOR APARTMENT AT 75TH
Street and Fifth Avenue in New York City.
While watching television one night, you hear
what sounds like a lion's roar. Well, there aren't any
lions around there, so you say, "It sounded like a
lion's roar, but somebody must have knocked some
garbage cans together, or a truck backfired. It's almost
impossible for that to have been a lion." You put it in
probabilities and say, "It's a million to one there's no
lion." You can use that low figure because it did
sound like a lion.

Out of curiosity, you go to your back window. It's
pretty dark, but you catch a glimpse of something
large jumping over the fence. It looked too big to be a
dog, but it couldn't be a lion. It must have been a dog.
Now, with this extra piece of information, you drop

the odds from a million to one to a thousand to one. Now you're curious, and go into the backyard with a flashlight. You find tracks that would take one heck of a large dog to produce. The combination of the roar, large figure, and large tracks makes you reassess the probabilities. You say, "Either I'm crazy, or there is a realistic possibility that was a lion," and you change the probability to a hundred to one against a lion.

The next morning, you pick up the paper and see an article on the front page with the headline, "Circus Comes to Town." Still thinking about the lion, you say, "By golly, the circus came to town," and you drop the probability to ten to one against the lion. A subtitle says, "Lion Escapes," and you change the probability from ten to one against a lion to a hundred to one there was a lion in your backyard. The next sentence says, "While the circus was going down Fifth Avenue around 76th Street, a lion escaped." Now, it's a million to one there was a lion in your backyard.

This shows how, starting from one end of a probability, fact after fact can change the probability, and it can swing almost 180 degrees in the other direction.

It's the same with the drug phenytoin. When it was synthesized in 1908, the probability that the medicine would be useful for eighty or more symptoms and disorders might have appeared to be one in a billion. There had never been anything like it. But, when the clinical evidence had been published by thousands of independent physicians (let me stress the word *independent*—they had no common interest other than to help others) in forty-eight countries, written in twenty different languages, and a host of basic mechanism studies support the clinical evidence, the odds that phenytoin is a broadly useful substance becomes astronomical. And the notion that it's only an anti-convulsant is absurd. But that's how it's listed with the FDA.

If a remarkable medicine is out of patent and sells for pennies, and no company deems it worth its while to go through the arduous and expensive procedures to get it approved by the FDA, should our public suffer?

The answer is simple. Was the FDA established just to prevent the negative, or was it established for the health of the American public? It was certainly the later. Action by them could correct a great catastrophe.

13. THE RULES
OF EVIDENCE

THE RULES OF EVIDENCE HAVE SOMETHING IN common with the Laws of Gravity. Neither can be amended by Congress or by any branch of government. The Rules of Evidence are simple. They are the application of common sense to probability.

Now, let us apply the Rules of Evidence to the question of whether or not phenytoin is useful for thought, mood and behavior disorders. The material on which this exercise is based is found in the Thought, Mood and Behavior section of *The Broad Range of Clinical Use of Phenytoin*.

There are many kinds of evidence: studies with placebo, studies in which a drug is effective after other drugs have failed, and trials in which a drug is found effective—is withdrawn and symptoms return, reinstituted, and symptoms disappear; and clinical studies in which improvements are confirmed by laboratory means. All of these methods have been used in establishing PHT's effectiveness.

Before arriving at a probability figure for thought, mood and behavior disorders, we will define them, for these purposes, to be problems of excessive anger and related symptoms such as impatience, irritability, impulsivity, hostility and violence; excessive fear and related symptoms such as worry, anxiety, apprehension, depression; also uncontrolled thinking, occupied by negative thoughts and interfering with concentration.

(In four papers PHT was not found "significantly" effective—not necessarily ineffective. For these purposes we allowed the four papers to eliminate ten positive papers that we have assessed the chance of being correct in one in two.) To arrive at an overall probability figure of PHT's usefulness for thought, mood and behavior, we assess individual probability figures to each of the studies. This is done by estimate, but since most of the authors assess the chance of their own work being correct in excess of 19 to 1 or 99 to 1, the following estimates are conservative:

Probability that
PHT is effective

	1 in 2
	1 in 2
	1 in 2
For each of the first seven reports,	1 in 2
controlled by phenobarbital and/or bromides,	1 in 2
we assess the probability of being correct of	1 in 2
1 chance in 2.	1 in 2

Lindsley and Henry, the first paper in
    non-epileptics, in problem children   1 in 2

Brown and Solomon, in delinquent boys   1 in 2

Silverman, in a jail study, 64 prisoners,
    double-blind crossover, placebo
    —also other drugs   5 in 6

Bodkin, observations of 102 nervous patients   3 in 4

Goodwin, 20 patients out of 20
    nervous patients   2 in 3

Walker and Kirkpatrick, 10 behavioral problem
    children out of 10, all improved   2 in 3

Zimmerman, 200 children with severe behavior
    disorders, 70 percent of cases improved   3 in 4

Cho, Sexton and Davis, 296 children,
    response rapid, often striking   4 in 5

Jonas, in his book, *Ictal and Subictal Neurosis*
    162 patients—over 12 years   3 in 4

Lynk and Amidon, 125 delinquents   3 in 4

Dreyfus, 80 patients   1 in 2

Rossi, behavioral problem children   1 in 2

Turner, 46 of 56 adult neurotic patients   2 in 3

Tec, 15 years' experience   2 in 3

Boelhouwer, et al., 78 patients, double-blind
    crossover and placebo   4 in 5

Baldwin, 109 children with behavior problems 3 in 4

Stephens and Shaffer, double-blind,
    30 adult outpatients   4 in 5

Goldberg and Kurland, double-blind,
    47 retardates, ages 9 to 14   3 in 4

Daniel, aged patients   1 in 2

Bozza, 21 slightly brain-damaged
    retarded children   1 in 2

Alvarez, in a book covering 25 years'
    experience   5 in 6

Stephens and Shaffer, second double-blind
    with 10 patients   3 in 4

Maletsky, episodic dyscontrol, 22 adults
    —other drugs had failed   3 in 4

Maletsky and Klotter, episodic dyscontrol,
    24 adults, double-blind with placebo 4 in 5

Solomon and Kleeman, 2 cases episodic
dyscontrol   1 in 2
Bach-Y-Rita, et al., 130 adults with assaultive
and destructive behavior   3 in 4
Kalinowsky and Putnam, 60 psychotic
patients, improvement in over half   1 in 2
Freyhan, 40 psychiatric patients, behavioral
problems   2 in 3
Kubanek and Rowell, double-blind, 73 psychotic
patients unresponsive to other drugs   4 in 5
Haward, double-blind, 20 psychotic patients   3 in 4
Haward, three double-blind studies: 3 in 4
concentration—last study, 59 pilots   3 in 4
Smith and Lowrey, 20 adult volunteers,
double-blind—cognitive function   3 in 4
Smith and Lowrey, 10 aged adults,
double-blind crossover—cognitive function   2 in 3
Stambaugh, hypoglycemia, unresponsive
to dietary management—including 6-hour
glucose test   3 in 4
Wermuth, et al., double-blind crossover,
19 "binge eaters"   2 in 3

Based on the foregoing, the chance that PHT is useful for thought, mood and behavior disorders is:

8,453,784,125,030,400,000 to 1.

PHT's parameters of safety have been established over a sixty-six-year period, by millions of people taking it daily, for long periods of time. It has properties which, viewed together, set it apart from other drugs. It acts promptly, calms without sedation, energizes without artificial stimulation, and has beneficial side effects. PHT is not habit-forming.

Conclusion—Having PHT listed in the Physicians' Desk Reference (PDR) only as an anti-convulsant is a grave injustice to the American public.

14. SUBSTANTIAL
EVIDENCE

IN THE FEDERAL FOOD, DRUG, AND COSMETIC ACT, the FDA is required to have "substantial evidence of effectiveness." The word "substantial" in this context cannot mean quantity. A study of 10,000 cases could be inconclusive. The evidence from a few cases can be "substantial." Let's take one example of how the evidence from just eight cases could be substantial.

For the purposes of this example, we eliminate the possibility of collusion, or hoax.

Suppose there is a government station in North Carolina that is set up to receive reports of UFOs. On average, they receive one call a day. Suppose that one night, between 3:00 and 3:10, eight calls come into this station, all reporting similar observations: to wit, that a huge ball of fire was seen slowly floating a few hundred yards overhead and suddenly, at tremendous speed, went upward and disappeared from sight.

Remembering our premise that collusion is eliminated, what are the probabilities that this really happened?

Since one call a day at random times is the average, the first call at 3:00 a.m. means no more than any other call received by the station. The second call could have been a coincidence. However, because it was within a ten-minute span of the first, this coincidence would occur, on average, once in 144 days (there are 144 ten-minute spans in twenty-four hours). The third call would be one heck of a coincidence: one hundred and forty-four times one hundred and forty-fourths of a chance. By the eighth call, the odds that there had been an unusual occurrence around 3:00 a.m. would be:

1/144 x 1/144 x 1/144 x 1/144 x 1/144 x 1/144 x 1/144 x 1/144 or 184,884,258,895,036,000 to 1.

This is "substantial evidence."

Now, in this UFO example, we took a premise that we couldn't take in real life, that collusion, or hoax, was impossible. The fact is, collusion would seem far more likely than anything else, and the investigators of this matter would spend a lot of time proving or disproving this.

We now come to the real-life proposition, the evidence that phenytoin (or PHT) is a widely versatile medicine. Here, the probability of collusion is ruled out by applying common sense to the facts.

Let's look at the facts before we apply common sense. Physicians in at least forty-eight countries have reported PHT to be useful for more than eighty symptoms and disorders, in over 350 medical journals, written in twenty different languages. Since the average physician receives seven or eight medical journals (less than a quarter of one percent of the world literature), it's obvious that the reporting physicians could not know of the work of more than a few of their colleagues. Common sense rules out collusion. Thus, the probability that PHT is a widely versatile drug is of the same order of magnitude as the UFO example.

15. MATHEMATICAL EVIDENCE THERE IS A GOD

WHEN WE SPEAK OF EVIDENCE WE SPEAK OF probabilities. Some probabilities can be figured exactly. The chance that you can call the toss of a coin correctly is one in two. To call it correctly twice in a row is one-half of one-half of a chance, or one-quarter of a chance.

There are probabilities that can't be figured exactly, only estimated.

If you were going to the phone to call a friend you hadn't spoken to in three months, and the phone rings and it's him, this is a long shot. You can only estimate the probability of it happening.

Let's go back to probabilities that can be figured exactly.

In January, Joe Smith bets a dollar in a lottery, and wins a million dollars. Joe had a million-to-one shot occur.

In February, Joe bets a dollar, and wins another million. The chance of this happening twice in a row is one chance in 1,000,000,000,000. Joe is on international television.

In March, Joe bets a dollar, and gets the same results. The odds are now 1,000,000,000,000,000,000 to one. The police put Joe in jail while they look for his accomplices.

Let's take a series of long shots that exact figures can't be put on.

A young man, Jack Dreyfus, won the City Golf Championship of Montgomery, Alabama, twice before he was twenty. He won seventeen club championships at four different country clubs, and qualified for the National Amateur three times out of three.

When he was fifty, he stopped playing golf. When he was sixty-one (with a great partner) he won the U.S. Open (amateurs and professionals) Lawn Tennis Championship for sixties and over. When he was seventy in Australia, with the same partner, he won the World's Open Doubles Lawn Tennis Championship for seventies and over. Jack was not a professional athlete. It's probably a hundred million to one against this. Let's use the conservative figure of a million to one.

When he was twenty-eight, he qualified for the Master's Bridge Tournament. When he was thirty, he devised a scientific method for playing gin rummy and beat the best players. *The Encyclopedia of Bridge*, for forty years, said he was reputed to be the best gin rummy player in the United States. Let's estimate it's a million-to-one shot.

He bred racehorses. Twice, he received the Turf Writers' Award: "Best Breeder of the Year." He was head of the Horsemen's Benevolent and Protective Association, and he received the Fitzsimmons Award: "One Who Contributed Most to the Best Interests of Racing." He was elected a member of the Board of Trustees of the New York Racing Association. On two occasions, he was made Chairman, the only person who was Chairman twice, and received the Eclipse Award: "Man Who Did Most for Racing." It's reasonable to estimate that it's a million to one against such a career in racing.

Jack started a small brokerage firm. Business was poor and advertising was necessary. The budget was so small that he had to write the advertisements himself. He had no education in advertising. Competing against the best advertising agencies, his firm received a gold trophy from Standard and Poor's: "Best Advertising in Wall Street." It's reasonable to estimate it's a million to one against this.

A mutual fund was started which Jack managed for twelve years. It got the best record of all the funds. We won't put a figure on that. He wrote the prospectus and did the promotion. He received an award: "One of the Five Best Marketing Persons for the 1960–1970 Decade." The odds against this are tremendous. However, let's just call it a million to one.

The head of research for Polaroid recommended that Jack buy the stock because they were making 3D glasses, and he did. 3D movies didn't succeed, but this brought Jack's attention to the Polaroid camera. He figured if it had come first, Eastman Kodak would have had a hard time selling its camera. So, he bought a lot of stock and made a tremendous amount of money. A close friend, Secretary of State William Rogers, estimated he was one of the fifty richest men in the country. (There was only one billionaire at that time.) As a boy, he hadn't made a go of three jobs at $15.00/week. His parents thought he would never make a living. Yet, he became one of the richest men in the United States. This is certainly a million-to-one shot.

Then, something important happened.

After suffering from an endogenous depression for over five years, Jack had ideas about electricity in his body, and asked his physician to let him try a drug not known to be useful for his symptoms. It worked, promptly. Over the next year, he introduced six people with similar conditions to physicians to receive the drug; they all had similar responses. For a patient to ask his physician for one drug out of a pharmacopoeia of thousands, and be correct, is unheard of; a billion to one. Let's just call it a million to one.

The chance of one man having seven million-to-one shots occur is one in 1,000,000,000,000,000,000,000, 000,000,000,000,000,000,000,000.

After unsuccessful attempts to get the medical profession to investigate, Jack felt obligated to leave his highly successful businesses in Wall Street to research the medicine, and established a medical foundation.

Over the years, the Dreyfus Medical Foundation discovered this medicine had been reported useful for over eighty symptoms and disorders by independent physicians around the world, in 350 medical journals, written in twenty different languages. The Foundation condensed these studies into bibliographies—one in 1970, one in 1975, and a third in 1988—and sent them to all the physicians in the U.S. The third bibliography contained 3,100 medical references and was accompanied by a book, *A Remarkable Medicine Has Been Overlooked*, which Jack wrote.

As shown earlier, it was a 1,000,000,000,000,000,000,000,000,000,000,000,000,000,000-to-one shot against Jack doing all these things on his own. There must have been a God that helped him.

AFTERTHOUGHT

That was written several years ago. It made a lot of sense to me, but I wasn't quite convinced. I've had some time to think about it, and now I am convinced. I've thought of two more "million-to-one shots" that I didn't include.

In the early stages of my trying to bring the phenytoin story to the government, I met with Secretary of Health John W. Gardner in 1966. He was nice and gave me some good advice. I told him that I thought our brains were like dry twigs that sometimes got on fire, and that phenytoin was like a gentle rain that calmed the fire. He laughed, and suggested I get a more sophisticated terminology.

An amazing thing happened two weeks after this. I came into my apartment, and on top of the sofa I saw a copy of a *Scientific American* book *opened* to two pages of a discussion on medical terminology on the brain, by Sir John Eccles. A friend had been sending me *Scientific American* for ten years, and I always put it on the coffee table. How this book got opened to the page I needed and displayed on the sofa, I'll never know. It was certainly a million-to-one shot.

Twenty-four years ago, my farm manager, Elmer Heubeck, called me on the telephone and said he thought they were going to have racing in Texas. He had a friend who knew of a beautiful 1,400-acre plot of land with limestone and oak trees that would make an ideal horse farm. It cost $450,000, and Elmer wanted to buy it but couldn't afford it. He asked if I would buy half of it with him. I agreed and put up $225,000.

We thought it unfortunate that racing did not start in Texas. However, our "farm" turned out to be one of the richest pieces of oil land in Texas. That was twenty-four years ago, and Elmer and I still get about $50,000 a month from the oil on this property. This was certainly a million-to-one shot.

This means that, if I had conducted my life on my own, the figure would be one chance in 1,000,000, 000,000,000,000,000,000,000,000,000,000,000, 000,000,000,000,000.

Thank you, God.

Mostly due to the Dreyfus Foundation's efforts, phenytoin is now being used in Brazil, Bulgaria, Cameroon, China, Dominican Republic, El Salvador, Ghana, India, Indonesia, Jordan, Lesotho, Lithuania, Mali, Mexico, Nigeria, Poland, Romania, Russia, Tanzania, Ukraine, and Zambia for a multitude of symptoms and disorders, including topical uses.

Although phenytoin was discovered useful in the United States in 1938, it's still only listed with our FDA for a single disorder. This is a catastrophe.

PART THREE

Worcester County Jail Study

16. THE EFFECTS OF PHENYTOIN ON EXCESSIVE FEAR AND ANGER

IN 1966, DR. OSCAR RESNICK AND I CONDUCTED a jail study on the effects of PHT with eleven prisoners at the Worcester County Jail in Massachusetts. It was done on a double-blind crossover basis.

In the study it was observed that the eleven prisoners had many symptoms in common that responded to PHT. Among these symptoms were: restlessness, irritability, fear, anger, inability to concentrate, poor mood, lack of energy, sleep problems, and an overactive brain. The results were exceptional, as you will see from the following quotes (taken from audio recordings) from prisoners themselves. All eleven prisoners showed improvement.

This jail study was to be an unusual experience for me—in some ways, the most fruitful of my life.

ACTUAL QUOTES BY PARTICIPANTS

DAVID

BEFORE DILANTIN	AFTER DILANTIN
I yell; I hit; blow my top; punch the wall; break something. I couldn't control it. I have a temper.	Calmer; haven't felt better; relaxed; I can control it; I forget it. [Dilantin] helped me physically, mentally, and emotionally.

JOHN A.

BEFORE DILANTIN	AFTER DILANTIN
Fly off the handle; tension; irritable; arguments in my mind; anger.	Much more relaxed; feel a lot better; more easygoing; still angry, but now I have a set of breaks.

ROBERT H.

Before Dilantin	After Dilantin
I get mad fast; get mad at myself; feel like taking something and breaking it; very edgy.	Contented; good frame of mind; no bad thoughts; I didn't have any run-ins.

WILFRED M.

Before Dilantin	After Dilantin
Very quick-tempered; pace the floor; nervous; blow my top; a lot of arguing.	More relaxed; I don't get in as many fights; more calm; I'm not so hot-tempered; my mind is more at ease.

ALBERT G.

Before Dilantin	After Dilantin
Quick tempered; fly off the handle; I get mad—start shaking.	Calm; relaxed; don't feel as much tension; haven't gotten angry.

JAMES D.

BEFORE DILANTIN	AFTER DILANTIN
Had a grudge; taking it out on everyone; I was getting into trouble. There was nothing but anger in me.	Kidding around; I'm not the same; I feel better; no more grudge.

DANIEL D.

BEFORE DILANTIN	AFTER DILANTIN
I can get pretty mad; wound up tight; blow my top.	Full of laughs; I'm relaxed.

CLIFFORD C.

BEFORE DILANTIN	AFTER DILANTIN
High-strung; things bother me; I let everything build up inside me; in a fight I can't control myself.	I feel wonderful; relaxed; good mood; I don't feel angry; I feel happy.

JAMES L.

BEFORE DILANTIN	AFTER DILANTIN
Miserable; a bunch of nerves; my thinking is bad; I'm down right now.	I feel a lot better; I ain't the same guy; I've been kidding around.

PHILIP B.

BEFORE DILANTIN	AFTER DILANTIN
I am quite nervous; too much on my mind; I've been very depressed.	I feel good all over; I relax a lot more. I feel good, very good.

VICTOR M.

BEFORE DILANTIN	AFTER DILANTIN
I have anger; I'm nervous; I don't sleep, pain in my stomach.	I'm in a good mood; I'm not as grouchy; I'm sleeping better; and the pain has stopped.

PART FOUR

Experiences

17. MOTHER

MY MOTHER WAS A SWEET WOMAN. ONE DAY, she and her sister, Bertha, were driving from New York to Montgomery, Alabama. After about 150 miles, they stopped at a roadside restaurant for lunch. Mother had to walk around the front of the car. As she passed the grille, she saw the usual gnats and moths to be expected there and exclaimed, "My goodness Bertha, can't you be more careful?"

When Aunt Bertha told us this story we laughed at the idea of her driving down the highway dodging moths and other bugs. Years later, it occurred to me that it showed how sweet my mother was. She even worried about little bugs.

Mother loved me, which wasn't always easy; I loved her, which was always easy.

18. APTITUDES

I LACK MANY APTITUDES. MY SENSE OF DIRECTION is in backwards. My copying device is faulty. My ability to remember names is so bad it's embarrassing. And I have a mechanical I.Q. of about seven. One good aptitude I was born with is a sense of probabilities.

My aptitudes to forget names and get lost I inherited directly from my father. Let me illustrate Dad's ability to forget names.

Dad, my wife Joan, and I were taking a train to Ocala, Florida. Hobeau Farm was being built by my farm manager and friend, Elmer Heubeck, and his lovely wife Harriet. On the train we drilled Dad. Every couple of hours we'd have him repeat, "Elmer and Harriet, Elmer and Harriet." We arrived at Hobeau Farm and went to a trailer to have lunch.

Dad walked in and said, "Hello Elmer. Hello Harriet." And Joan and I were proud.

Harriet has a pet name for Elmer. She calls him Abbie. During lunch she would say, "Abbie, may I have some coffee?" "Abbie, please pass the butter." Abbie this, Abbie that.

Dad couldn't stand it any longer. He said, "I know this is Elmer. I know this is Harriet. But why does she keep calling him Chuck?"

19. THE CONCORD

I'VE KNOWN FOR A LONG TIME THAT I HAVE A small ego. One night, I got what I call objective proof. I'd gone to the Catskills to vacation where no one knew me. The Catskills are a couple of hours from New York; I was driven up there to a hotel called the Concord. The Concord has a dining room that is about as large as the average farm. It might be four or five acres in size. With my sense of direction, if I was hungry, I'd better start out half an hour early to find my table.

Everybody was assigned a waiter. I had a young fellow about eighteen or nineteen years old. A good description of him would be to say that he was, "aggressively indifferent." I gave him large tips all the time. Sometimes, I came to breakfast late, and he would say, "The kitchen is closed." I'd see other people getting apples or peaches and I would ask, "Well, couldn't I get an apple or a peach?" and he'd say, "Oh, sure," and he'd get it, but he never volunteered.

One night, I found my table in only ten minutes. I ordered the roast beef. By the way, you could get any amount of food you wanted. You could get roast beef and chicken the same night. I ordered the roast beef and got a small round piece; it was pretty tough. I worked on it for a little while; finished about two-thirds, and still felt hungry. I said to the waiter, "The roast beef I had was pretty small. May I have another piece?" He said, "Yes," and went into the kitchen and came back with a humongous piece of roast beef. Just looking at it discouraged me, and I realized that I wasn't as hungry as I thought. I didn't want the roast beef; on the other hand, I realized I would look like a jackass for asking for more roast beef if I didn't eat at least some of it. There was a dilemma: put something in your stomach you didn't want, or look like a jackass. At least that's what I thought.

There was a large menu on my table. One side of it was blank. I thought this won't do any harm: I tore the menu in half, took the blank side and, when no one was looking, put the roast beef in it, folded it up and put it in my jacket pocket. Then, I put my hand in my pocket and the package felt damp. It was a new suit so, when nobody was looking, I took the other half of the menu and rewrapped the roast beef. Now, it was sort of moisture-proof. I finished dinner and left. When I got about fifty yards away from the scene, I saw one of those trays where they put the leavings. When no one was looking, I put the roast beef there and kept going.

Nothing registered with me until a few days later; then I thought, this is funny. How many people would be that concerned about an indifferent eighteen- or nineteen-year-old boy? How sensitive can you be? You really have a small ego. You knew you had a small ego, but now you've caught yourself and got objective evidence.

20. SLOP OR GARBAGE?

DURING THE WAR, I SERVED IN THE COAST Guard. It was felt, with my college education, I would probably be competent to collect garbage. So, I was assigned to a garbage truck. I was third in charge, although I had the highest position on top of the truck. Garbage cans would be handed me by the second in charge, and I would empty them. At night, I could tell how good business had been. When I took my clothes off, there would be a brown line around my stomach, or chest, depending on the haul.

It was while I had this fine position that I learned the difference between garbage and slop. The difference is simple. Slop is slop. Garbage is slop with coffee grounds.

This information should make you glad you picked up this book.

Never leaving the base became an awful bore. I would have given anything just to walk through a grocery store. Some of the fellows were beginning to say dumb things, like they wished they could get into the fighting. But one day I got off the base. The three of us had a good load of garbage and were ordered to bring it to the Mineola garbage dump. Not far from Mineola people started waving wildly at us. We thought, "How wonderful." We'd heard how much people appreciated the uniform, but had never experienced it. The people waved, and we waved back, and felt patriotic.

We were enjoying this when a car, with the words "Fire Chief" on it, pulled alongside. The driver gesticulated for us to stop. We stopped—in the center of Mineola. Then we noticed we had a load of burning garbage. The chief ordered us to dump it, and we did. Firemen came, put out the fire, and shoveled the remains back into our truck, and we took it to the dump. On the way back to the base nobody waved at us.

21. FURTH BURNER

GOING FROM GARBAGE TO PSYCHOLOGY, WE all have observed that we don't like to be caught without knowledge. There's no use admitting you don't know something, if you can get away with it. I have noticed this in the medical profession. Dr. Green will say to Dr. Brown, "As you know Hempleworth and Snodgrass, in 1924, showed that eels have more cholesterol than sardines." Dr. Brown may never have heard of that paper, but he's not apt to let on. This is human. I saw it in the Coast Guard.

The canteen, where you bought everything from candy bars to clothing, was oblong and almost the size of a football field. At the entrance, there were many telephone booths so you could make phone calls. Then you went through a door into the canteen. Once you got into the canteen, you were not allowed to go back through that door. One day, it was raining hard. I was inside the canteen when I remembered a phone call I'd forgotten to make. I didn't want to go outside and make that long trip in the rain to get back to the phones. So, I tried a maneuver—I don't know where I got the nerve. I approached the guard at the entrance door and started to go through. He said, "Where do you think you're going, Mate?" I said, "It's okay, I'm a furth burner." He said, "Oh," and I went through. That was fun. I did it a few times when it wasn't raining just to keep my spirits up.

One day, a guard was at the door who was less ashamed to show his ignorance. When I said, "It's okay, I'm a furth burner," he said, "What's a furth burner?" I said, "Where do you think they get the hydrocarbon in the canteen?" That was different, and I went through.

22. SUMMA CUM ORDINARY

At Lehigh University, where I was graduated Summa Cum Ordinary, I tried to get good grades, but I didn't kill myself. I must be on the dumb side because I got straight "C's," with one exception. I got an "A" in Music Appreciation.

Professor Shields was playing Cesar Franck's *Symphony in D Minor* in class. I was taking a light nap, hoping it would be mistaken for music appreciation. At one point, Professor Shields stopped the music and said, "Dreyfus, what do you think of this music?" I woke up and said, "It's inexorable."

I'd never used that word before or since, and I don't know where it came from. It probably wasn't in

Professor Shields' immediate vocabulary either, because he gave me an "A."

Ever since then Cesar Franck's *Symphony in D Minor* has been a favorite of mine. I recommend it for your listening.

PART FIVE

Conclusion

23: THE FDA

THE FDA WAS ESTABLISHED, IN THE BEST
tradition of good government, to help
American citizens in matters of health, in ways
they can't help themselves. But it was conceived as a
defensive unit. If it were a football team it would have
six tackles and five guards, and no one to carry the
ball. All that was expected of the FDA was defense—
to protect us from dangerous substances and unwar-
ranted claims of effectiveness.

Understandably, the founding fathers of the FDA
presumed that the drug companies, with their profit
incentives, would furnish the offense. It could hardly
have entered their minds that a drug company would
leave a great medicine "lying around." Nor would
they have been able to figure out how to equip the
FDA against such an eventuality unless the FDA were

put into the drug business, which is a far cry from the original premise—and is not being recommended here.

The FDA has done nothing about PHT. This is to be expected when a drug company doesn't play its role. Unfortunately, this does not leave the FDA in a neutral position. Through no fault of the FDA's, PHT's narrow listing has a negative effect. Absence of FDA approval is thought of by many as FDA disapproval—or at least as a sign that something is lacking. The system of drug company through FDA to physician has become such a routine that the physician, with other things on his mind, waits for the system to bring him PHT. It's been a long wait.

The real purpose in establishing the FDA was to improve the health and well-being of the citizens of the United States. The neglect of a great drug certainly falls into that category. If a man were drowning and a doctor had prepared to throw him a life preserver that had more lead than cork, the FDA would say, "Hold it! That thing might hit him and kill him, and even if it doesn't it can't help him." Nice work, FDA. But suppose the FDA knew there was a good life preserver under a tree, which the doctor didn't see. Shouldn't they say, "Try that one, Doc"? Of course they should.

It is not suggested that the FDA go into the drug business. It is more than suggested, in this extraordinary case, where thousands of physicians have furnished us with many times the evidence required to get approval of a new drug (keep in mind this drug has been approved for comparative safety and has stood the test of over sixty years of use), that the FDA should no longer take a hands-off policy. It's a sure thing our public shouldn't suffer any longer because Parke-Davis stayed in bed after Rip Van Winkle got up.

Let us understand the magnitude of what we're talking about. The non-use of PHT has been a catastrophe. We are not accustomed to thinking of the non-use of a medicine as a catastrophe. We think of a catastrophe as a flood, a famine, or an earthquake, something tangible, overt, something in the positive tense. But something passive, such as the non-use of a great medicine that can prevent suffering and prolong lives, is also a catastrophe.

Something must be done. How it is done is for the government to decide. But here is a suggestion. It would seem a waste of time, and thus to the disadvantage of the American public, for the FDA to attempt to approve the many clinical uses of PHT separately. That could take forever. It would be far simpler for the FDA to address itself to the basic mechanisms of action and give PHT a listed indication-of-use as a stabilizer of bioelectrical activity, or as a membrane stabilizer. Certainly the published evidence for this is overwhelming. Such a listing would stimulate the physician to think of clinical applications of PHT and to refer to the existing medical literature.

Even a nod from the FDA to the physician would help. It could take the form of a letter to the physician, calling attention to the literature of his colleagues, and reminding him that since PHT has been approved for safety he is permitted to use it for whatever purposes his judgment suggests. Certainly the FDA would never try to tell the doctor how he should use PHT. That's always the doctor's decision. But such a letter would lift the cloud of negativism, and the physician would get an unobstructed view of PHT and the work of his colleagues.

I'm sure the problem–agriculturists will say that if the FDA takes any action in this matter it will set a precedent. Fine. Good. If this happens again, if another established drug is found useful for eighty or more disorders by thousands of physicians, then the FDA should take this as a precedent.

Every once in a while, routine or no routine, a little common sense should be permitted. This is an extraordinary matter, vital to our health. If the FDA was set up to help the American public, here's a chance to do something great for them—with no one's feelings being hurt except routine's.

24. A UNIQUE PRIVILEGE

WHAT HAPPENED TO ME DOESN'T HAPPEN IN real life. I took Dilantin on a hunch. You just don't ask your doctor to let you try one drug out of a pharmacopoeia of tens of thousands, and find it works. Yet, this is what happened.

After I took Dilantin, my good health returned. I was neither tranquil nor ecstatic. I was just all right. For the first time in my life, I realized how good you feel when you feel "all right."

I got out of a depression by finding a drug that had been overlooked. Could Dilantin help others as it had helped me? It seemed highly improbable. How could an important medicine have been overlooked for twenty years? It didn't make sense; but if it were so, I had an obligation to do something about it.

This gave me a unique privilege—to spend my money, and the last forty years of my life, trying to get the information to the rest of humanity.

I can't imagine a nicer life.

25. TO THE PRESIDENT
AND TO CONGRESS

ALTHOUGH THIS MATTER IS NOT YOUR CONVEN-
tional work, please don't think it's not one of
the most important matters ever to come
before you. Look at it this way. This is a not a problem. This is a solution for some of our most serious
problems.

The most versatile and benign medicine ever given
to us is listed with our government agency for only
one use. And the reason—it's so cheap. Think of that.

For God's sake—and I do not use His name in
vain—shouldn't the President and Congress set up a
committee of intelligent and conscientious people to
study this matter? It would only take a week or ten

days. And the rewards for the American people would be inestimable.

Jack Dreyfus

is the author of four books.

The fourth book, *The Story of a Remarkable
Medicine*, contains a summary of the relevant
material of the first three books, and a summary
of their success.

The Story of a Remarkable Medicine can be
found in bookstores, on www.amazon.com, and
at www.remarkablemedicine.com